ESSENTIAL OILS AND AROMATHERAPY

The Elixir of Longevity

ESSENTIAL OILS AND AROMATHERAPY

Copyright © 2017

Disclaimer

All the material contained in this book is provided for educational and informational purposes only. No responsibility can be taken for any results or outcomes resulting from the use of this material.

While every attempt has been made to provide information that is both accurate and effective, the author does not assume any responsibility for the accuracy or use/misuse of this information.

Essential Oils and Aromatherapy

The Elixir of Longevity

NATHAN WAKE

Table of Contents

INTRODUCTION

Our world is surrounded by heavenly scents; scents that can raise a dampened spirit, scents that can excite a depressed soul, scents that can calm a fraying nerve and scents that can equilibrate a distracted mind. These scents are found in the petals of flowers, in the leaves of grasses, in the bruises of trees and in the roots of plants. All around us, nature beckons on us to heal our bodies, to heal our spirit, and to do so with a smile, with faces wrapped in the pleasure of beautiful fragrances.

It is amazing to realize that healing can come from our breath, and this has little to do with respiration, but everything to do with the perception and inhalation of pleasant scents. It is glorious to know that there are some medicines that you do not have to squeeze your face to take as, from certain appealing fragrances, a perfect health can be achieved. This is the backbone of the whole concept and practice of aromatherapy.

Thus, aromatherapy is delineated as the art of using plant constituents, essential oils and those derived from aromatic plants, distilled from plant leaves, fruits, roots and barks, moss and animals to foster all-round well-being. The practice of aromatherapy has far-reaching importance, ranging from its application in complementary medicine to its utility in conveying certain emotional or psychological benefits like relaxation and sensuality, as well as respite from stress and nervous tension.

The use of aromatherapy extends to different aspects of our lives. For example, the feeling of relief on perceiving the scent of a jasmine in full bloom during a stroll on a cool summer evening; or the inexplicable feeling on perceiving the aroma of hot cinnamon buns fresh from the oven while walking past a local bakery.

In effect, when an aroma stimulates a feeling within us, be it nostalgia, euphoria, relief, sensuality, etc., then there is aromatherapy at play, and this is achieved by utilizing the power inherent in the fragrance of plants.

By employing one or a blend of the over four hundred essential oils within the therapeutic arsenal of aromatherapy, psychological as well as physical benefits, as well as total wellness spent in long life, is inevitable.

This is the true *Elixir of Longevity!*

CHAPTER ONE

The History of Aromatherapy

Aromatherapy dates back to over 3500 B.C., inexorably linked to the advance of aromatic medicine, which in early times was itself fused with magic and religion.

In ancient Egypt, incense prepared from aromatic woods, herbs and spices were also burned in veneration of their deities, believing that their prayers reached up to the heavens as incense rose. However, aromatics paved the way for the introduction of aromatherapy. Essential oils such as cinnamon, ginger, myrrh and sandalwood were employed by ancient civilizations in medical treatment.

In fact, around 2650–2575 BC, embalming was carried out by the Egyptians in their quest for immortality, while Frankincense, myrrh, galbanum, cinnamon, cedar wood, juniper berry and spikenard have all been employed by the Egyptians at certain historical points for the preservation of the bodies of their kings in preparation for the life yonder. A pharaoh's dead body was always gorged with a mix of palm wine and the herbs of Chamomile and Galbanum.

The essential oils of these herbs and spices were arduously transported through unfriendly routes and dry deserts by Arab dealers for delivery to Assyria, Babylon, China, Egypt, Greece, Rome and Persia. Frankincense and myrrh are believed to have been the most besought materials, and had a value that was equivalent to gems as well as precious metals, due to their high demand which surpassed supply in those early days.

Perfumery

Apart from their application of fragrances in the sphere of religion, the Egyptians, especially the wealthy ones, were famous in their penchant for schematizing simple fragrances into their everyday lives, such as inclusion of perfumed cones by women as a part of their habiliment – cones which would melt under the heat to release their enchanting fragrance. Also, to protect their bodies from the desiccating effects of the scorching desert sun and to restore the beauty of their skin, Egyptian women traditionally anointed their skin with sweet smelling oil.

Ancient Papyri discovered in The Egyptian Pyramids told of the application of essential oils in the management of every kind of illness, not very different from present day applications.

During 1539–657 BC, the practice of refining aromatics in cosmetics, medicine and perfumes. In fact, up till some centuries preceding Jesus Christ's birth, the perfume industry of the Egyptians was renowned as the most excellent in all of the Middle East and the lands beyond. Their reputation as leading perfumers was so prodigious that, in celebration of Julius Caesar's return with Cleopatra, bottles of perfumes were thrown into the cheering crowd in demonstration of his complete conquest of Egypt.

Even before this time, the use of plants as medicine was common knowledge. Our forefathers scented woods and burnt aromatic herbs to expel and exterminate 'bad spirits' from the infirmed.

In China, Shen Nung, a Chinese practitioner, wrote the book *Yellow Emperor's Classic of Internal Medicine* around 2697 BC. A book which has entries on the properties of more than three hundred different plants, as well as their uses in medicine, suggesting that the Chinese might have been first aware of the knowledge of plant-based medicines. This is the most ancient surviving medical book. In addition, even though the Indians and the Americans also employed plants as medicines, Chinese documentaries remain the most comprehensive evidence. Chinese civilizations, in addition, perfected the application of essential oils and herbs.

Within that same period, the Egyptians advanced the practice of aromatherapy. Aromatherapy, as practiced by them, was akin to that of the Chinese; that is extracting botanical materials and burning woods that possessed scents to pay homage to gods.

Meanwhile, during the preceding 1,000 years, the people of Hebrew, Assyria and Babylon, among others, had already embraced the wealth of knowledge hidden in Egyptian *botanical pharmacopoeia*, due to their profound knowledge of aromatic medicine. So much so that, by the time the Egyptian Empire crumbled, Europe had taken up the gauntlet, championing the art of empirical medicine, where novel practices steadily evolved into an orthodox scientifically medical system.

Also, ancient Greeks excelled in their application of essential oils, applying them both in medicine and cosmetics. Asclepius was the first known Greek physician and lived and worked in 1200 BC. He employed the combined use of herbal materials and surgery with a skill the like of which had never been previously seen, and so great was his reputation that he was immortalized in Greek mythology as the god of healing, with several temples which were called *Asclepieion* raised in homage to him.

Hippocrates, who lived around 460–377 BC, the father of medicine, was the earliest physician to do away with the Egyptian tenet that illnesses were triggered by forces beyond the natural. He instead was of the opinion that a physician should find likely causes of diseases by carefully examining and observing the patient, arriving at a conclusion only after evaluation of the signs. Hippocrates's methods of treatment typically involved little physio-therapies, as well as baths. He also favored massaging the patient using infusions, as well as the employment of certain herbs such as fennel, parsley, hypericum or valerian for internal use.

More than a millennium ago, a Greek physician known as Pedacius Dioscorides published a manuscript on herbal medicine, in which he prescribed many remedies, most of which are still very much in use in aromatherapy.

Furthermore, the expansion of the empire of Rome into Greece and Egypt brought Romans in contact with the medical knowledge of some of these advancing civilizations, expending and expanding on their knowledge of the discipline of aromatherapy. And with the incursion of the Roman Empire into Asia, and the establishment of a newly growing trade route, novel oils became introduced into Europe from India, China and Arabia.

1000 AD was a landmark in the development of aromatherapy as Avicenna, a physician, became the first to include the distillation process in the distillation of the essence of rose. In Arab world, it was during this time that alcohol was first distilled with its combination of essential oils to produce the first perfumes.

The Spanish invasion of North and South America brought new plants and oils in contact with Europe. The quantity of therapeutic plants found in Incan, Mayan and Aztec plant gardens, including the wealth of knowledge in their possession concerning the application of these botanical materials in healing, was amazing to the Spanish. The North and South Americans had their own recipes for herbal remedies, and were very conversant with the application of essential aromatic oils especially in medicine and religious ceremonies.

It is not, however, until the initial periods of the 19th century that European scientists started studying the action of aromatic oils on humans.

French chemist, Gattefosse, had a laboratory accident in which he burnt his hand and immersed it in lavender oil. He was impressed at how quickly the hand healed upon treatment with the essential oil and, in the year 1937, he released a book that centered on the anti-microbial properties of oils. He is accredited with the first usage of the word 'aromatherapy'.

Dr. Jean Valnet was a French medical doctor and, in 1964, fascinated by Gattefosse's research, started investigating the application of aromatic oil in medical treatment by applying it on patients in his clinic. Margaret Maury, enthralled by Dr. Valnet's research, applied Valnet's findings into her beauty therapy, tailor-making beauty treatments to achieve customer specificity, and proceeded to set up the earliest aromatherapy clinics in France, Switzerland and Britain, applying essential oils in fostering vibrant, youthful skin, which today is referred to as the day spa.

Aromatherapy, in recent times, draws more patronage than ever before. In addition to its use in medicine and in the home, there are so many spas in different parts of the world which cater for people of different backgrounds and inclinations. Spas serve as a place of solace, where stressed out working men and women go to be bathed, massaged, and wrapped in recipes that have their origins in civilizations long past, like the Egyptian, Roman, Grecian and Oriental civilizations, taking the story back to where it began.

CHAPTER TWO

Essential Oils

The term 'essential oil' is generally employed in the categorization of concise conveyance of natural, volatile, aromatic fluids that comprise Essential Oils, CO2s, Absolutes and Resins.

'Essential oil' as a term is a contraction of 'quintessential oil', which came from the idea advanced by Aristotle that there are four components of matter – fire, air, earth and water. The fifth element, also known as the quintessence, was believed to be the spirit of matter, which could be released upon distillation and evaporation. This idea is reflected in our usage of the term 'spirits' to describe alcoholic beverages like whiskey.

Today we know that, contrary to this primitive belief, essential oils are physical in nature as a complex combination of various chemicals. They are strong liquid extracts, generally distilled from plant parts such as leaves, seeds, flowers, bark and stems, among others by the use of steam or water.

Essential oils come in a wide range of colors and consistencies, like some which are clear with watery texture, to the thick, syrupy and dark ones. They are generally of very high concentration and should be used in small quantities.

Absolutes

Absolutes are aromatic liquids of very high concentration, distilled from plants using chemical solvents which are withdrawn in the final steps of extraction, leaving behind a highly concentrated essence.

Absolutes are produced for several reasons, one of which is that the distilling of a plants essential oils by steam has a lot of setbacks, such as limited extraction of the essential oil constituents, and because steam extraction sometimes breaks down the valuable natural oils that are contained in delicate flowers. Just as is the case with essential oil extracts, absolutes have to be used as a matter of necessity, with care, respect and knowledge.

One notable difference between essential oils and absolutes is that while essential oils, in the hands of properly trained personnel, can be taken internally to great benefits, absolutes generally are avoided for internal use because they contain traces of the solvents used in their extraction.

CO2s

These are are oils extracted by the use of the supercritical CO_2 (carbon dioxide) method.

In its natural state, carbon dioxide exists in gaseous form, and this is the form used in respiration. Carbon dioxide, however, can be compressed into liquid state, which acts as a solvent capable of liquefying the natural components present in plant material. Following extraction, the CO_2 returns to the natural gaseous state, leaving behind the resultant extracts known as CO_2s.

CO_2 extracts possess a potential benefit over essential oils because there is no risk of damaging the constituents, as opposed to the steam distillation of essential oils.

CO_2s are categorized into two, namely:

CO_2 Selects

CO_2 Select are extracts produced when low pressure is employed in the liquefaction of the CO_2. CO_2 Selects contain the volatile (aromatic) components of the plant materials that are capable of dissolving in liquefied CO_2. Each aromatic molecule has its own molecular weight, and some happen to be too heavy to remain in steam distilled essential oils. However, CO_2s can solubilize these heavy constituents, hence, CO_2 extracts are often more viscous and have an aroma closer to the smell of the natural herb.

CO_2 Totals

In the production of CO_2 Totals, a far higher amount of pressure is employed. CO_2 Totals contain all or almost all of the elements capable of dissolving in the liquefied CO_2. CO_2 Totals are generally more viscous than CO_2 Selects because they contain more than just the volatile constituents of aromatic CO_2. They also contain lipids, waxes, and other components capable of solubilizing in the pressurized CO_2.

Resins

Upon sustaining an injury, certain plants produce a thick, sticky and sometimes solid substance known as resins. Some examples of resins include frankincense and myrrhand benzoin. The commercial production of some resins may require that the tree is injured in several places to enhance its ability to produce resins.

Natural resins confer medicinal benefits though they prove difficult to work with in aromatherapy. For example, it is difficult to work with benzoin resin because of its extremely thick and sticky nature.

Tears of frankincense are small, solid pieces of frankincense resin. Both the resins of frankincense and myrrh come in solid form and, traditionally, are not applied in their resinous form within holistic aromatherapy. They are usually powdered and applied for medicinal use.

The essential oils of frankincense and myrrh are steam distilled from the resin for employment in holistic aromatherapy, religious, room fragrance and perfumery.

Carrier oils

Carrier oils are oils employed in the dilution of absolutes and essential oils before using them on the skin. Carrier oils are generally used with two purposes in mind:

- To act as a vehicle, conveying the essential oil unto the skin
- To reduce the concentration of potent oils before application by serving as diluents

In contrast to essential oils, which are generally volatile and possess concentrated scents, carrier oils are less volatile and do not evaporate, imparting their scent less strongly than essential oils. Avocado, peanut, sweet almond, pecan, wheat germ, apricot kernel, grape seed, olive, etc., are examples of carrier oils.

CHAPTER THREE

Methods of Production and Use of Essential Oils

It is astonishing for people when they first realize that, to produce a little quantity of essential oil, you need several kilograms and tons of the botanical material. For example, to produce 1kg of rose oil, you need 2,000kg of rose petals. In fact, to obtain 1kg of jasmine absolutes, you need approximately 4 million jasmine flowers! Hence, it is clear that a lot of time and resources go into the production of essential oils. This is because essential oils are the 'spirit' of a plant; its essence.

Essential oils are known to offer both mental and physical advantages when applied in the correct manner. Hence, it is important to know what essential oil is and what it is not. For instance, artificial, chemically-based replications of essential oil which do not have any health benefits are often included in perfumes to retain the fragrance and extend the time during which it can remain viable for use. These, you should keep in mind, are not essential oils.

A few of the processes involved in extracting essential oils from various parts of botanical materials are as follows:

Steam Distillation

In the production of essential oils by steam distillation, the producers obtain the potent oil extracts from precise plant parts such as the leaf, the root, the bark, the berry or the flower. To do this, a still is arranged into a system and packed with botanical material. Steam produced by boiling water in another part of the system is made to suffuse the botanical materials, turning the volatile components of the plant matter into vapor. The vapor is then passed through a cooling chamber where it is regained in a liquid state by condensation. The oil thus obtained is what is known as essential oil. They are usually of very high concentration, with different parts of the plant yielding different quantities of oil, which is also reflected in the pricing.

Cold Pressing

Cold pressing is usually employed for the 'expression' of essential oil from the peels of fruits like lemon, orange, lime and grapefruit. The oil obtained from cold pressing is usually more bountiful than that produced using steam distillation, making the price of essential oils obtained via cold press much lower and reasonable.

Enfleurage

Enfleurage is a process used in the extraction of scents that is employed mainly on the flowers of plants. This is achieved by placing the flower on a cloth or any material that is capable of trapping the essential oil. The blossoms are changed on a daily basis with new flowers until the absorbent material becomes saturated, following which it is squeezed to release the extract. The essential oil obtained is usually not pure, coming in a combination of waxes and resins.

Alcohol Extraction

Some plants like Jasmine, gardenia and narcissus are capable of releasing their scents when placed in an alcohol or like solvent preparation. Absolutes is the name given to the resulting extracts.

General Uses of Essential Oils

Physical and Psychological Uses

As has been mentioned several times before, apart from the physical use of essential oils, their application in influencing mental dispositions are very notable. To achieve this, you have to inhale the diffused oils. However, responses to each particular oil vary depending on the individual's inclination and the memory the scent is associated with. For example, someone who associates jasmine with the memories of the joys of childhood would have a different response to the scent from someone who associates it with a heartbreak. Apart from their ability to evoke memories, however, the oils possess innate chemical properties that confer on them their ability to stimulate, or soothe, or create an equilibrium. For example, lavender is ambivalent in its effects, calming in small quantities but exciting when applied in larger doses.

As Cleaner

In addition, when applied to clean the home essential oils are less toxic, and a more pleasant substitute for commercial products. For example, using a few drops of an antiseptic oil like orange, lemon or eucalyptus, in the ratio of 10% essential oil to 90% water, to clean sinks, bathrooms and other appliances would provide as much utility as commercial detergents, if not more.

Beauty Products

Essential oils are also very useful as cosmetic products. They find use in hair products, as well as products for skin and bathing. There are a lot of products that you can produce using essential oils, to the extent that you can make your own face and body lotions, cream lip balms, etc.

Insect Repellent

A myriad of essential oils like peppermint, lavender and citronella have been employed as natural insect repellents. To achieve this, massage diluted oil into the skin as you would suntan oil. You may also prefer to use a spray bottle. In this case you have to add your essential oil blend into the bottle and use it as you would insect spray. Another way to use essential oils as an insect repellant is to add it to your burner so that the scent can pervade the air and keep insects away.

Simple Equipment Employed in Using Essential Oils

Diffuser

For the psychological application of oil, you would need to diffuse or spray the oil into your surroundings, hence you would definitely need a diffuser. An excellent 'air pump type' diffuser will disintegrate the molecules of the essential oils into tiny particles, making it easier to inhale. It is bad practice to put oils on light bulb rings because the thermolabile components would be destroyed by the heat generated by the ring, causing it to lose its ability to heal.

Humidifiers

It is common practice for people to use humidifiers in the dispersion of essential oils into the air. This makes sense except that, if you use a humidifier made of plastic material that does not have a chamber made specifically for oil, you may run the risk of destroying your humidifier because essential oils tend to attack many types of plastics.

Burners

Some diffusers come as burners and, even when they are quite cheap, are really very aesthetic, although they are generally not as effective as the air pump type diffusers. You might want to choose one that has an appropriate space for the inclusion of a candle, as well as an oil compartment. This will stop the oil from getting toasted.

Other methods

Another method of employing essential oils is to introduce some drops into a spray glass bottle containing about 90–97% water, 1% natural emulsifier and 3%–10% essential oil. The emulsifier is introduced to reduce the surface tension between oil and water and to enable them to mix. Note, however, that the percentages of the different components might be determined by the purpose of use as well as the setting. For example if you are in a bathroom, you might opt for a higher oil ratio in the mix. Do not fail to properly shake the bottle before use, as the oils will not be properly distributed in the mix and would be used up in one spray if it is not well shaken, since it will float to the top of the bottle.

In employing this kind of spray, avoid spraying the mix at anyone because the oil might precipitate allergic reactions in sensitive skins. Excellent oils that can create nice sprays include orange for revitalization and spearmint to create a balance.

CHAPTER FOUR

Effective Use of Some Notable Essential Oils

There are several available essential oils but the ones listed below could be said to be so invaluable that they can constitute an initial kit for anyone who is interested in taking up aromatherapy.

Bergamot Fruit Peel *Citrus bergamia*

You can diffuse bergamot fruit peel into the air to raise the spirit, as well as to pacify minor instances of anxiety. In Earl Grey tea, bergamot fruit peel is responsible for the uplifting orange-like note.

Uses

Its application is mainly topical, on the skin, used for acne, chicken pox and shingles. The fragrance is very delectable, and appreciated by many people, as it serves as a delightful fragrance when sprayed in rooms.

Cautions and Contraindications

- Bergamot fruit peel oil is phototoxic, so it is not recommended to be worn in the sun, as it may lead to the irritation of sensitive skin.
- It is also not recommended for internal use.

Chamomile, Roman Flower *Chamamelum nobile*

Roman chamomile oil has a healing effect, and is applied for its soothing effect on the nervous system, as well as a restorative nature which provides a calming effect on many people.

Uses

Roman chamomile is a great oil for skin use, tightening the skin tissues and enhancing its puffiness. It also possesses anti-inflammatory activity, hence, it might work well for burns, inflammation of the skin and eczema.

Roman chamomile oil is also useful for pain due to its analgesic effect. It is also good for sleeplessness, insomnia, or premenstrual symptoms as well as in meditation. Roman chamomile is a bit costly, but that is because of its far reaching importance.

Cautions and Contraindications

- Roman chamomile should be avoided in the first three months of pregnancy.
- In addition, if you have any form of allergy to ragweed, be very careful when using Roman chamomile so as to avoid allergic reactions.

Eucalyptus globulus Leaf

Eucalyptus globulus is the most common and widely-preferred variety of eucalyptus.

Uses

Eucalyptus globulus has the smell of camphor, and is applied in conditions affecting the respiratory tract, such as inflammation of the sinus, inflammation of the bronchi, and lower respiratory tract infections, like infection of the lungs, etc.

Applying a little quantity to the skin might help muscle aches and pain and, in addition, help to relieve fever. In fact, it may be beneficial when diluted with water and used as spray for menopausal hot flushes.

Eucalyptus globulus has an anti-bacterial property and may decimate the bacterial population by up to 80% by simply spraying it into the air. Hence, in disinfecting your home, you might find *Eucalyptus globulus* very useful. It is also useful for disinfecting fabrics by dropping in water – not the fabric. It should not, however, be used on sensitive fabrics.

Cautions and Contraindications

- You should avoid instilling eucalyptus oil into children's nostrils. Eucalyptus globulus can be very dangerous when misused. For instance, 3.5ml when consumed, whether internally or via absorption into the skin, can lead to death.
- You should also avoid using eucalyptus oil in children.
- Avoid using with pregnant women.
- It is also contraindicated in hypertensive and epileptic patients.

Frankincense Resin *Boswellia carterii*

Besides myrrh, frankincense is another traditional yuletide oil, proving that this oil has been around with us a long while, since even before the birth of Christ. This reflects how valuable they are. Along with frankincense, gold and myrrh were the most treasured substances, fit to be given as a gift to the Messiah.

Uses

The oil of frankincense has a long history related to its anti-infective property. The gum from the tree is extracted by steam distillation. It may be employed in skin application if you have skin that is not prone to allergic reactions. You can establish your sensitivity status by doing a patch test on the base of your arm.

The oil of frankincense has an anti-infective property and may improve aeration by fostering deeper breathing.

In the beauty industry, the use of frankincense mainly boarders on its use for dry, aging skin. When used on scars, wrinkles and stretch marks, it has an impressive effect. Furthermore, you would certainly be better for it if you employed frankincense in a diffuser to reduce anxiety, and improve meditative practices.

Cautions and Contraindications

- In pregnancy, avoid the use of frankincense.
- It is also not meant for internal use.
- Epileptic patients should not use frankincense.

Geranium Rose Leaf *Pelargonium graveolens*

Just like its close relative, Chinese geranium, Rose Geranium is extracted from leaves of *Pelargonium graveolens*.

Uses

Rose Geranium is brilliant when applied for many skin conditions like oily skin, acne, burns, eczema (both the dry and the weepy variants) as well as for itching and dermatitis. It has a triple action, being anti-fungal, anti-bacterial and anti-inflammatory. It helps in skin decongestion and improves the elimination of skin toxins. This is because it maintains a balance in skin oil production, and helps in the regeneration of cells, thus serving as a panacea for the skin.

For psychological application, Rose Geranium is good for the relief of nervous tension and peri-menopausal symptoms, as well as pre-menstrual syndromes. The plant has a flowery scent, with a distinct note that is rose-like, positioning it among the best choices when you are looking for an excellent mid note in perfume blends. It is among the most important oils to include in your kit.

Cautions and Contraindications

- Rose geranium should be avoided in the initial stages of pregnancy.
- It is not meant for internal use, so you should do well to avoid such usage.

Ginger Root (Fresh) *Zingiber officinalis*

Made from the steam distillation of ginger rhizomes, Ginger is a commonly used spice.

Uses

It is excellent when employed as a blend in muscle aches and poor circulation. Hence, using it in a diffuser for respiratory conditions like flu, inflammation of the bronchi and cough.

Ginger oil has an emotionally stimulating effect. Hence, it might be good for depression. You can also use it to reduce nausea and bloating by diluting it in a vehicle and applying on the stomach.

Cautions and Contraindications

- Ginger may irritate an allergic skin, and the root is mildly phototoxic.
- Do not use ginger oil in babies and in the first three months of pregnancy.

Juniper Berry *Juniperus communis*

Juniper berry oil is extracted by steam distillation from the ripe berry, and juniper oil is amenable to all skin types in terms of provision of relief.

Uses

To use for beautifying purposes, it is recommended that you make a facial steam with the oil extract of juniper berry. This could be applied in the treatment of oily skin with blackheads, psoriasis, stretch marks, weeping and infected eczema, etc. It is also good in the treatment of inflammatory conditions, stiff joints and in gout. Traditionally applied as a decontaminant, possessing the ability to detoxify a room when diluted to a potency of 5% and sprayed into the air.

Cautions and Contraindications

- Juniper berry oil is contradicted in pregnant women, breastfeeding mothers and babies.
- It is not meant to be used internally.

Lavender Flower *Lavandula officinalis – L. angustifolia*

Lavender oil is the most commonly sold essential oil. Made from the steam distillation of the leaves and flowers of *Lavandula officinalis,* it is recommended if you plan to capitalize in the sale or distribution of essential oil.

Uses

Lavander oil helps in cell regeneration, and is also good for burns. The first step is to cool the burn with ice, or cold water, followed by the application of the lavender oil on the affected area. Lavender oil has a wide range of uses and can be helpful fpr pain and skin damage, as well as many other skin conditions like acne, dermatitis, eczema, insect bites, stings, rashes, rosacea, sunburn, wounds, burns and blisters. It can also balance sebum and prevent scars.

On a mental level, lavender is employed for its calming effect on the nerves, and organic lavender is specially employed for this. Furthermore, lavender in low doses acts as a sedative, but acts as a stimulant in high doses.

Other properties of lavender oil, such as its analgesic effects, makes it an excellent succor in pain. It is also useful as an anti-inflammatory, anti-infectious and restorative agent.

Cautions and Contraindications

- Lavender, in contrast to most essential oils, is amenable to the straight application onto various skin types. However, it should be diluted before application in people whose skin are sensitive, as it can produce inflammation in such people.
- Avoid usage in the first trimester.
- Lavender should not be used internally.

Lemon Peel *Citrus limonum*

Lemon peel oil is obtained by cold press extraction of the peel of *Citrus limonum.*

Uses

Lemon peel oil finds use in the preparation of formulas for blond hair, due to its lightening effect on skin pigment, as well as its ability to maintain the hair's flaxen tones. Lemon also improves and fosters the shine and growth of the hair respectively. In cellulite, pimples, boils, dry skin, etc., lemon is of very great importance. The health and strength of hair and nails, as well as the maintenance of equilibrium in the secretion of sebum, improvement of epidermal strength, toning of the blood vessels, etc., are all parts of the beneficial effects derived from the use of lemon oil.

To the mind, lemon is a stimulant, aiding in the maintenance of constancy of thought.

Cautions and Contraindications

- Similar to many oils produced from fruit, lemon can be phototoxic; therefore you are advised not to wear the oil in the sun.
- In addition, do not use lemon if you are sensitive to it.

Lemongrass *Cymbopogon citratus*

The oil of lemon grass is extracted by the steam distillation of *Cymbopogon citratus.* Largely underutilized, lemon grass oil is a very pleasant oil, and proves to be more dynamic with its lemony fragrance than straight.

Uses

Lemongrass essential oil is useful as an anti-inflammatory agent. As an antiseptic and restorative, it is also very useful. In cosmetics, oily skins, acne and cellulite respond well to lemongrass. Because of its antiseptic effect, it could be used as a cleaner for homes and floors, as used in Indonesia.

Psychologically, lemongrass has a soothing effect on the nerves and hence serves as an excellent soporific.

Cautions and Contraindications

- Lemongrass can irritate the skin and so its use should be avoided in allergic patients.
- Lemongrass should not be used in pregnant women.
- Its use internally should be avoided.

Manuka Leaf *Leptospermum scoparium*

To make manuka leaf oil, the leaves and end branches of the plant are extracted using steam distillation. It is an anti-infective which in New Zealand has found use in the treatment of fungal, bacterial and worm infections. It is also useful in muscle aches, and vaginitis and proves, as an anti-infective, to be more effective than tea tree in clearing some certain bacteria and fungi that prove to be resistant.

Cautions and Contraindications

- Manuka leaf oil is a taboo for pregnant women.

Melissa Leaf and Flower Lemon Balm *Melissa officinalis*

Melissa is extracted by steam distillation from the leaves and flowers of the *Melissa officinalis* plant. It, however, a difficult oil to extract because of its low yield, making Melissa not just exorbitant to purchase, but rare and precious.

Uses

Melissa proves to be very useful in the management and treatment of Herpes Simplex (cold sores), with the best effect obtained when the oil is applied before full eruption, during the itchy phase. In the same vein, bee and wasp stings are well managed using Mellissa oil.

In addition, Melissa may be used as an antihypertensive and to reduce palpitation. Because of its soothing effect on the central nervous system, it may be used as an anxiolytic, as well as in the management of premenstrual syndromes.

Cautions and Contraindications

- Melissa causes allergy in sensitive skin.
- Its use should be avoided in glaucoma.
- It also is not meant to be used internally.
- It is contraindicated in pregnancy.

Myrrh Resin *Commiphora myrrha*

Myrrh resin is distilled from the hard gum resin of *Commiphora myrrha*.

Uses

Myrrh is traditionally employed to prevent skin-aging, ulceration, fungal infection, and weeping eczema as well as wrinkles. In dental health and eczema, myrrh finds an excellent application. Adding a drop in water helps to heal the gums.

Cautions and Contraindications

- Myrrh is a very viscous and sticky oil, and hence should not be added to nebulizers as it will clump them up.
- Also, since myrrh has a very strong fragrance, when making a Christmas blend, it is recommended that a smaller quantity of myrrh be used with frankincense to prevent its strong scent from over-powering the mix.
- Myrrh in large doses can be toxic.
- Its use is contraindicated in pregnancy and breastfeeding mothers.

Orange Bitter Peel *Citrus aurantium var. amara*

This essential oil is obtained from the cold compress of the peel of the fruit of *Citrus aurantium*.

Uses

Bitter orange finds its use in cosmetics so as to strengthen and soften pale, dry, smutched or crinkly skin. It has also been used to rekindle nerve endings, to rehydrate a dry skin, moderate oil secretion and aid cell regeneration.

When diluted and formulated as a rub, bitter orange oil serves as an excellent soothing agent for aching muscles. Adding it into a diffuser makes it amenable for use with cold, flu, anxiety and sleeplessness.

Cautions and Contraindications

- Bitter orange peel is phototoxic and high doses may be allergic to the skin.
- Its use should be avoided in the first three months of pregnancy.

Peppermint Leaf *Mentha piperita*

Peppermint oil is extracted by the steam distillation of the flower of this plant obtained at the flowering stage. There is a lot of information on peppermint as a great deal of study has been done on it, having been around in European culture for many centuries. Peppermint is ubiquitously available in several products made for domestic use, such as toothpaste, gum, teas and room fresheners.

Uses

In aromatherapy, peppermint is an oil of many uses and has a far-reaching importance. It is employed in the treatment of shingles and acne and is also used as a decontaminating agent. It is also useful when capillary vasoconstriction is desired. Peppermint reduces itches and rashes, and generally is a good anti-inflammatory agent.

When diffused into the air, it has a decongesting effect and has a capacity to excite the mind. 5ml in a diffuser, mixed with 95ml of water, can be sprayed into the air to keep the mind attentive while performing tasks or during study.

The oil also has analgesic properties, and can be used for bruises when the skin is not broken, as well as for headaches.

Cautions and Contraindications

- Peppermint should not be used in pregnant women and lactating mothers.
- It can cause contact dermatitis in some people.
- Avoid introduction into the eye and nostrils.
- Peppermint is not meant for internal application.
- Do not use in neonates and infants. This should be avoided to the extent that a diffuser containing peppermint oil shouldn't be sprayed near babies and infants, as it may lead to reflex apnea and spasm of the larynx.

Ravensare Leaf *Ravensara aromatic* (Cineole)

The oil of ravensare is obtained by the steam distillation of the leaves and branches of *Ravensara aromatic*. In terms of smell, it has a fragrance that is very similar to that of eucalyptus.

Uses

The oil obtained from Ravensare Leaf is an immune booster, and is also employed for sinusitis, respiratory conditions and muscle ache. It has an antiviral effect that makes it very useful in the management of chicken pox and shingles, for which purpose it is diluted in a vehicle, usually an oil (5%) and applied with a clean brush.

It is very effective when used against flu, colds and inflammation of the bronchi.

Cautions and Contraindications

- Avoid use with pregnant women and breastfeeding mothers.
- It is not meant for internal use.
- It should be noted that, while sometimes this plant is called Cinnamonium camphora, Ravensare and Cinnamonium camphora are quite different plants. And while there may be a mix up about the oils, always ensure that the label bears Ravensara aromatica.

Rose Otto Flower *Rosa damascena*

This essential oil is obtained from the steam distillation of the flowers and the even so, the yield is so low that it takes about seventy whole flowers to produce just a single drop of the oil. Rose oil has a singular, compelling scent which makes it widely enjoyed by humans.

Used

It is employed in the treatment of dry, aging and sensitive skin, as well as creases and eczema. It also helps to heal broken small blood vessels and in hormone regulation. Rose oil has been used as an astringent, as an antiseptic and as an anti-inflammatory agent. Generally, rose oil has a stimulating effect on the nervous system.

Cautions and Contraindications

- Rose oil is contraindicated in the first three months of pregnancy.
- In individuals with sensitive skin, rose oil should be used with caution or avoided altogether as it can irritate the skin of such individuals.

Rosemary Leaf *Rosmarinus officinalis*

When the leaves and flowing tops of rosemary are steam distilled, the resulting oil is the rosemary oil, a wonderful oil that is present in many shampoos, especially shampoos made for dark hair.

Uses

Rosemary has traditionally been employed in the treatment of spots on the skin, oily hair and dandruff. Rosemary is agreeable to the hair, and is thus an invaluable oil to include in shampoos and hair conditioners. By adding about 10 drops to a 100ml glass bottle of natural shampoo, and shaking well, rosemary can promote hair growth within rational anticipations.

By diffusing and breathing rosemary oil, mental acuity could be achieved, as rosemary has a stimulating effect on the mind. Hence, like peppermint oil, rosemary is favored when there is mental work to be done, offering improved concentration.

Cautions and Contraindications

- Rosemary may cause an upsurge in blood pressure and hence should be avoided in hypertensives.
- In addition, rosemary oil may precipitate allergic responses on skins that are sensitive.
- It should be avoided in pregnancy.
- Epileptic patients are also advised to avoid rosemary oil.
- Avoid use in neonates and infants.

Tea Tree Leaf *Melaleuca alternifolia*

Tea tree oil, a very popular essential oil, extracted by the steam distillation of the leaves and branches of *Melaleuca*. It has been used in several products, including toothpaste, soap, etc.

Uses

Tea tree oil is effective in dermal conditions like abscesses, eruptions, cold sores, dandruff, infections of the skin, stings from insects, warts and pimples. As an antiseptic, tea tree oil has a broad spectrum of activity and is cidal to a wide range of bacteria. It is also used to repel insects.

Tea tree oil is an essential part of your aromatherapy kit if you want to have one. Sometimes, companies generate different lines of product using this singular oil.

Cautions and Contraindications
- Tea tree oil can irritate a sensitive skin, and so should either be applied with caution in such skin or avoided totally.
- In high concentration, it is also toxic.
- Avoid use in pregnant women.
- Finally, do not use tea tree oil internally.

Yarrow Leaf and Flower *Achillea millefolium*

This essential oil is extracted by the steam distillation of the aerial parts of the *Achillea millefolium* plant.

Uses

Use the oil for acne, burns, eczema, varicose veins and scars. It has great utility when applied to foster hair growth, as well as maintaining equilibrium in oil secretion by the skin and the scalp. Yarrow has a blue hue due to chamazluene. It is this particular component that is responsible for the curative and revitalizing property of the Blue German Chamomile. Yarrow oil encourages sweating and acts as an excellent antiseptic, anti-inflammatory and anti-allergenic substance, with analgesic properties.

Cautions and Contraindications

- Do not use yarrow oil during pregnancy.
- Avoid in neonates and infants.

CHAPTER FIVE

The Art of Blending I

Blending in Perfumery

Just like culinary skills and processes, aromatic blending can stick religiously to a recipe without straying or diverting from the laid down steps. It can also be done at liberty, in which the ingredients are substituted for other ingredients of choice, as well as being completely radical, allowing you to upturn every known recipe and lose yourself to the direction of a creative mind. When a blend is made, it is usually made for the sole purpose of its eventual fragrance, and even when therapeutic properties may come with the final blend, aroma and not therapeutics is its sole purpose.

Most modern perfumers think it is a difficult, if not impossible task, to design an excellent perfume from natural scents alone. They believe that chemically synthesized copies of natural essential oils are very necessary for the impartment of a complex dynamic to their scents. Hence, perfumes are made with as many as over a hundred chemical essence combinations to achieve a final blend.

This, however, is not necessary when you are working with natural essential oils because these, unlike their chemically synthesized counterparts, already possess in natural combination a lot of constituents. Consider rose oil, for instance; it has a combination of over three hundred constituents, which means that for a chemist to synthesize rose oil and blend with jasmine oil, for example, they would have to synthesize over four hundred constituents to arrive at an acceptable blend. Hence, it is an impossible task to synthesize identical copies of certain essential oils.

Furthermore, chemical synthesis of essential oils is never a great option because, with such a quantity of constituent synthetic chemicals, there is a high likelihood that these chemicals can precipitate allergic reactions in users.

Further to this, there are safety measures that you have to put into consideration when compounding any type of blend, including aromatic blending. For example, when you use bergamot, you want to be extra careful because of its phototoxic properties. In addition, you should keep away from using oils that should be avoided for a condition you have.

Perfumers who work in fragrance houses employ a great deal of their lifestudying and mastering the art of perfumery and, while many perfumers employ only essential oils as well as other natural ingredients, others, in order to cut costs and produce a more stable fragrance with a longer shelf life, harmonize a blend of both natural essential oils and chemically synthesized ones.

When blending for aromatherapy, however, we stick to the natural ingredients such as essential oils, absolutes, CO_2s, alcohol, carrier oils, herbs and water.

You will have to pay attention to the basic essential oil categories created on the basis of their aroma bases.

- *Essential oils based on flowers:* These include Lavender, Neroli, and Jasmine
- *Essential oils based on wood:* Here you find Pine and Cedar
- *Essential oils based on earth:* Include Oakmoss, Vetiver and Patchouli
- *Essential oils based on herb:* Are Marjoram, Rosemary and Basil
- *Essential oils based on Mint:* Here you find the likes of Peppermint and Spearmint
- *Essential oils based on Medicineare:* Eucalyptus, Cajuput and Tea Tree
- *Essential oils based on Spice:* Nutmeg, Clove and Cinnamon
- *Oriental Base Essential oils:* Are Ginger and Patchouli
- *Essential oils based on Citrus:* Include Orange, Lemon and Lime

By trial and error and with practice, you will become conversant enough with these essential oils to know blends that go well when combined and those that do not. Some interesting examples include: floral based essential oils, which make excellent blends when combined with essential oils based on spice, citrus and wood; wood based oils which make excellent blends with every category of essential oils; spicy and oriental oils which, when used with flower, oriental and citrus based oils are marvelous, as long as you remember to use oriental oils in very little quantities when you work with them; and finally, essential oils based on mint which produce amazing blends when used in combination with wood, herb and earth based essential oils.

Harmonizing Your Blend

Everyone who has ever used perfumes are very familiar with the fact that, many hours after a perfume had been applied, there is a side to the fragrance that is not the same with the initial scent. This is because some essential oils are more volatile than the others and hence evaporate faster. As these volatile oils are lost through evaporation, the remaining oils in the blend will change in reflection of the essential oils that are left.

Therefore, to be able to blend properly, you have to know your notes. The **top note** based oils are the most volatile essential oils in a blend, and are lost within one to two hours after application. They include: Anise, Grapefruit, Orange, Basil, Lavender, Peppermint, Bay Laurel, Lemon, Petiigrain, Bergamot, Lemongrass, Spearmint, Citronella, Lime, Tangerine and Eucalyptus.

The **middle note** based oils take a little longer, lasting between two and four hours before they are yielded up to the atmosphere as vapors. Examples include: Bay, Fir Needle, Rose, Bois-de-rose, Geranium Rose Geranium, Cajeput, Hyssop, Rosemary, Carrot Seed, Jasmine, Rosewood, Chamomile, Juniper, Berry, Spruce, German Linden Blossom, Tea Tree, Marjoram Common, Roman, Neroli Tea Tree, Cinnamon, Nutmeg, Clary Sage, Palmarosa, Thyme, Clove Bud, Parsley, Tobacco, Cypress, Pepper, Black Yarrow, Dill, Pine, Scotch, YlangYlang, Elemi and Fennel.

Finally, the **base note** oils last the longest, some lasting for several days before the fragrance is finally lost. Examples of base note essences are: Angelica Root, Frankincense, Patchouli, Peru Balsam, Ginger, Sandalwood, Beeswax, Helichrysum, Vanilla, Benzoin, Vetiver, Atlas Cedarwood, Myrrh, Cedarwood, Oak Moss, Virginian and Olibanum.

As has been mentioned elsewhere, while you might need to stick to some of the rules at the beginning, with greater experience in aromatherapy, you will realize that you may not really need to confine yourself to the rules. You might want to give room for boundless imagination and creativity. In the meantime, you might want to learn the rules like a novice so that you can, with greater experience, break them like a pro. Some of the tips to keep in mind include:

Rule 1

Any time you want to create a blend, begin by adding between five and twenty drops of the combined blend. This will help you to keep wastage of oil to a minimum if you later realize that you do not feel kindly towards the outcome of your intended blend.

Rule 2

At the initial stages of your blend, make use of pure essential oils, absolutes or CO2s only. This will prevent you from wasting any alcohol or essential oil if you find out that you do not like the blend or the fragrance you have created.

Rule 3

Keep a record of your better recipes, detailing drop by drop the amount of oil you employed in its creation, and of course the name of each oil essential oil you utilized. The reason for this is that it is not very difficult to forget the exact recipe for your blend, and one extra addition of oil to your blend could make all the difference to the outcome. Hence, once you have realized that one perfect blend, you want to guard it jealously by putting it on record. Otherwise, you might lose your precious recipe and the effort, time and resources employed in its creation.

Rule 4

With regards to storing your new fragrance, employ an essential oil vial or, if you like, a fancy perfume bottle, both of which are readily available and not difficult to find.

Rule 5

Never forget to painstakingly label your blend. Use codes to label the ingredients, not only to maximize space, but to keep your blend a secret.

Rule 6

There is an important rule of thumb in blending and that is to keep a good balance of your notes. A rule of thumb recommends 30% blend of top note essential oil, 50% of middle note oil, and 20% base note oil. Refer to previous sections of this chapter for the essential oils that you should employ both from the different categories and their different notes.

Rule 7

Never forget the concentration and potencies of your oils. Keep in mind that absolutes and CO2s possess higher concentration than essential oils, hence, except you want their scents to dominate the blend, you have to use little quantities of the more potent oils.

Rule 8

You will find it very useful if you invest your time in checking out the characteristic strengths of oils at different dilutions. This you can do by making a 20% dilution of the oil in carrier oil by adding a drop of essential oil to 5 drops of carrier oil, and studying the characteristic fragrance of that dilution. You may then add more drops of carrier oil to dilute further to a 10% dilution, and study the fragrance again.

Rule 9

The ninth and final rule is to allow your blend to age by leaving it to sit for a few days. You should also study the fragrance after this time because, most times, fragrance tends to evolve when combined and softens.

CHAPTER SIX

The Art of Blending II

Therapeutic Blending

In therapeutic blending we are more concerned with creating a blend that will help in alleviating a given psychological or physical condition, and more emphasis is placed on achieving therapeutic results and not necessarily on the fragrance achieved with the final blend. However, the good aromatherapist tries marry a therapeutic blend with an excellent fragrance.

When you are blending for therapeutic purposes, keep these three tips in mind.

Tip 1

Use oil because of ots ability to deliver therapeutic effects.

Tip 2

Ensure that the oils you are about to employ are free of side effects and are incapable of affecting other aspects of your general well-being.

Tip 3

Evaluate and remember the therapeutic actions you set out to achieve and eliminate from the mix any oil that will not advance this intended result. Let's illustrate with peppermint and cypress. Assuming you have created a blend of these two oils which you intend to take before bedtime for menstrual cramps, a closer look will reveal that the blend in itself is counterproductive to your intention because the oils' stimulating effect will prevent you from sleeping.

Refer to the previous chapter, following the same basic principles laid down there. There are a few other things to keep in mind.

Substituting Oils

There are more than two hundred essential oils, absolutes, CO2s and carrier oils at the disposal of an aromatherapist to work with and, considering that the prices of some of these oils are quite on the high side, you may sometimes find it necessary to substitute some of these more expensive oils. And, apart from financial reasons, there are several reasons why you might want to substitute some oil; sensitivity to some oils being a ready example.

If you realize that you do not possess all the essential oils required for the creation of a given aromatherapy recipe, you can try substituting with some of the essential oils at your disposal and, while the final aroma might be quite different from what you set out to achieve, a careful substitution may still get you a similar and practical result.

Aromatic Substitutions

In a recipe where your reason for substitution is really the final fragrance and not for any reason therapeutic, then you have to substitute essential oils from the same family of oils, like citrus or floral or spicy or earthy. If, for example, you are looking for a substitution of the essential oil of sweet orange, you might have to look for mandarin which provides a similar scent. If you want to make a substation for rose otto, you might want to go for rose geranium, which may not be a perfect substitution, but it will give you an approximate result at a more economical price.

Other possible substitutions include lime for lemon and vice versa, tangerine for sweet orange, neroli for ylang-ylang, peppermint substituted for spearmint, and cinnamon substituted for clove.

Making Therapeutic Substitutions

The rules in therapeutic substitution are quite different from those employed in aromatic substitution for, in therapeutic substitution, the aroma of the oil can be different in that it can achieve the same therapeutic result as well as produce a scent that is delectable to work with.

Therefore, you have to be very sure that the new oil you are going to choose will give the same result as the one you are substituting it for, while at the same time paying close attention to the side effects and contraindications.

CHAPTER SEVEN

Essential Oil: Storage and Safety Tips

Essential oils do not generally go rancid, but some oils lose their quality with age, deteriorating in terms of both fragrance and therapeutic effect. Some oils, for example citrus oil, with time begin to lose their aromatic and therapeutic properties to oxidation. Contrastingly, when stored well, some oils like sandalwood and patchouli possess more quality with time by looking mellow and spherical.

Nonetheless, to avoid loss of quality of your essential oil over time and to protect it from losing its aromatic and therapeutic properties, you should keep your oils in amber bottles, as this helps to protect them from sunlight which catalyzes degradation reactions. Storing essential oils in plastics is not a good idea, and is definitely not a good practice, as essential oils can dissolve them.

Finally, store essential oils in cool, dry conditions.

Safety tips in the use of essential oil

Essential oils are liquids of high concentration and, when misused, could produce harmful effects. This, however, does not cause unnecessary fear about the use of essential oil. Just remember to treat essential oils as medicines, following the safety tips outlined below. These tips are definitely not exhaustive, but it will go a long way and, if you encounter any difficulty in the application of essential oil in aromatherapy, you can consult your doctor or a qualified and trained aromatherapy practitioner.

Safety Tip 1

Never apply undiluted essential oils on your skin except lavender and tea tree oils. Even at that, do not attempt the application of any essential oil to your skin undiluted until you have acquired significant knowledge of essential oils and their use.

Safety Tip 2

Some individuals react when their skin comes into contact with some essential oils. Further to this, always do an initial skin patch test if you are about to use an essential oil for the first time. The test is quite simple. Place a little quantity of the diluted essential oil on the inner side of your elbow, then wait for twenty-four hours. If the oil does not cause irritation to you after this time, you may consider it safe for your own use. Keep in mind the fact that the absence of allergic reaction on your skin when you use an essential oil does not clear it for use in other people.

Safety Tip 3

Do not use essential oil without consulting your physician if you are pregnant, regardless of what the literature says. This is also true for other special conditions like hypertension, asthma, epilepsy, etc.

Safety Tip 4

When making use of essential oil, try to use the least amount that can achieve the result you are expecting. If a drop can get the job done, do not add an extra drop for the fun of it.

Safety Tip 5

Essential oils, like medicines, should be kept out of the reach of children. Don't be carried away by the pleasant scent of oils; always keep in mind that essential oils are medicines and medicines, in the hands of the inexperienced, are poison.

Safety Tip 6

Employ the use of essential oils only after you have sought extensive consultation from a qualified and trained aromatherapist.

Safety Tip 7

Essential oils, like most oils, are inflammable. Hence, you should keep them away from fire hazards.

CONCLUSION

Thank you for downloading this book!

Aromatherapy is such a wonderful field because, unlike many other medicines where health comes out of discomfort, out of pain, out of squeezing faces, and pained expression, aromatherapy offers healing conferred by beautiful scents and wonderful fragrances. Therapy administered amidst closed eyes and deep sighs, all in a bid to take a lungful of beautiful scents. There is power in our breath and there is even more power in the scents we take in with each one.

This book has tried as much as possible to foreground the ancient science and practice of therapy through aroma. It has tried to emphasize the many benefits that many people are only subconsciously aware of by shifting aromatherapy from the hands of some gifted few to the handd of anyone who craves absolute wellness and long life, and who want to partake in the healing that exudes from the bedrock of essential oils.

With this book, everyone can make simple blends of essential oils to achieve both aromatic and therapeutic purposes. My wish for you is that this book will help you *create that magical blend* of fragrances that can set you apart in the world and make you **live long in wellness**.

Thank you once again!